Paleo Diet For Beginners

———— ❧❧❧ ————

How Paleo Can Help You Lose Weight Quick With Fast And Easy Healthy Recipes

By Jennifer Sullivan

Free Gift

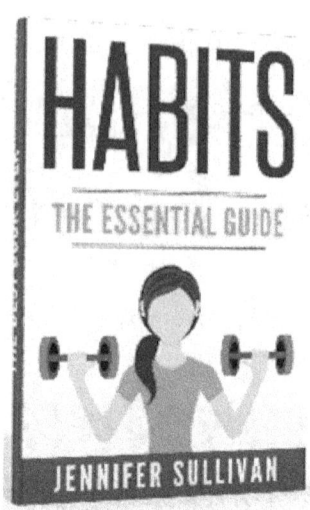

Discover The Secrets Behind How You Can Hardwire Your Brain for Success with Simple Habits!

Smoking, skipping breakfast, and procrastinating, these are some of the habits that we all know we should change and erase from our lives. However, even if changing these habits have been a part of your resolution list for so many New Years', it's still hard to let these habits go. Well, let me tell you that it is going to change now.

Not Everyone Wants to Admit It

To become the best, you must stop looking at the big picture and start working on the small yet important stuff—your habits!

>>Visite the URL Below To Download "Habits: The Essential Guide" For FREE<<

https://cueballpublishing.leadpages.co/free-habits-ebook/

Introduction

I want to thank you and congratulate you for purchasing my book, *"Paleo Diet For Beginners: How Paleo Can Help You Lose Weight Quick With Fast And Easy Healthy Recipes"*.

This book breaks down the building blocks of the popular paleo diet and how you can use it to your benefit to get the body you always desired! The main concept discussed in this book is that it is not only about the scrumptious and healthy recipes in a paleo diet but also it is important to adapt healthy and smart routine habits that will accelerate the effects of a diet.

Turning to our genetic makeup to unlock the causes of modern disease, a growing number of scientists now suggest that our genes are nutritionally tied to our prehistoric past. Are you tired of fad diets and compromises that don't seem to work with your genetics and cannot be sustained in the long term? If you've been struggling to find an eating regimen that supports lifelong health, helps improve physical fitness and promotes mental well being, the paleo diet might have the answers you've been looking for.

Based on the dietary habits of our stone-age ancestors, the paleo diet is a relatively new addition to the vast landscape of diets to become popular in the last few decades. As it rejects the pitfalls of the modern Western diet, the Paleolithic diet encourages the consumption of clean, natural foods that work with the body's genetic makeup and chemistry.

Thanks again, enjoy! ☺

The information herein is offered for informational purposes solely, and is universal as so. The presentation of the information is without contract or any type of guarantee assurance.

The trademarks that are used are without any consent, and the publication of the trademark is without permission or backing by the trademark owner. All trademarks and brands within this book are for clarifying purposes only and are the owned by the owners themselves, not affiliated with this document.

Table of Contents

Introduction 4

What Is The Paleo Diet? 8

    What Is Wrong With The Modern Diet? 10

    How Going Paleo Can Boost Your Health 13

    Eating Paleo Is Beginner-Friendly................................16

    Criticism And Different Interpretations.........................18

Paleo Essentials: What To Eat And What To Avoid 22

Staying On Track: 4 Key Tips To Keep Your Motivation Up..27

Paleo Recipes 30

    Salads..30

    Soups 41

    Main Dishes..51

    Sides/Vegetables...66

    Desserts 73

Before You Go 83

Conclusion..85

What Is The Paleo Diet?

It is said the existence of human beings spans longer than two million years. Our dietary conditions have changed vastly since then. Although partly due to evolution, we have experienced many of changes, but let us look back to 10,000 years ago. It is the time studies suggest the human race changed its dietary routine and food quality.

The concept of the paleo diet comes from 10,000 years ago, when our diet was aligned with our body gene requirements. In contrast to the Standard American Diet (SAD), the paleo diet helps us cut back the amount of sugar we excessively take in our daily life.

Therefore, sometimes referred to as the caveman or stone-age diet, the paleo diet is a natural, back-to-basics eating regime centered on consuming simple, fresh, and unprocessed foods, similar to what our ancestors ate in the Paleolithic era. It is a high-fiber, high protein diet, which reduces weight with cutting calories. As modern humans have increasingly relied on refined grains and processed goods, a host of health issues have emerged, which can be traced back to what we eat in the first place!

What our ancestors were used to eating in old days, which they hunted and found, can also be eaten by our generation. Paleo diet is the only way to provide us with long-lasting health benefits. This nutritional approach works with genetics to keep you more energetic and strong.

Many researchers in biology, biochemistry, ophthalmology, and dermatology determined the food we eat today is refined food, trans food, and sugar, which becomes the cause of diseases like obesity, diabetes, high blood pressure, infertility, depression, and other chronic illnesses that have been shown to correlate strongly with diets rich in sugar, refined gains, processed fats, salt and dairy products. Briefly, many of the staples of the modern Western diet are bad for human health.

As we look back on our ancestors, we find they were not only noticeably leaner, more athletic and more resistant to disease than we are today, but they also consumed high quality, natural foods. At the core of the Paleo diet is the idea that what you eat should work with your genes and your biochemistry to ensure optimal health!

The main concept of the Paleo diet, as discussed above, is to have natural and unprocessed food. The food involved in such a diet has high fat, low to moderate carbohydrates, and low animal proteins. In our normal diet, we look into calorie count a lot, but in Paleo diet, calorie count is unnecessary.

There are many reasons calorie count is discouraged in a Paleo diet. For starters, conscious intake of low calories helps in losing weight in the short-term, but it is likely that you gain as much weight as you have lost in the future. The reason is that taking less calories does not help in building an effective metabolism system, but is only a short-term solution for a weight watcher.

Paleo diet encourages to build a stronger and healthier body mechanism. This proves it as a long-term investment to our health. For adopting this diet, it is important to consume well-treated and freshly grass fed animals or wild fish or shellfish. The philosophy behind this is the same as to consume the same meat our ancestors had in our primitive times.

What Is The Paleo Diet?

The main purpose of adapting the Paleo diet is to invest in long-term and prosperous health. It is not only about what to eat and what not to, but it is a habit that involves how much to exercise, how much to sleep, and how to lead a proper and healthy routine.

It is not that hard to adopt a Paleo lifestyle. The major thing to focus on here is to be happy and light, not just physically, but also mentally. With a better working internal system, losing weight is definitely no problem.

What Is Wrong With The Modern Diet?

The advent of agriculture several thousand years ago marked a turning point for human civilization. It allowed us to settle down and build vast societies, but it also came at an unfortunate cost. The discovery of farming meant processed grains formed the basis of our diet.

Another problem is we are moving more toward artificial substance and machine-made things, rather than natural. We are also working 24/7 paying no attention to our healthy lives and eating food that only fills the stomach, but does not fulfill the body's requirement as needed.

Another harsh dilemma is that we are living on a pill, which boosts the system, and we think we are doing fine, but it is destroying our health. Machine-made, processed, canned foods cannot match naturals food our ancestors used to eat.

They didn't suffer from diseases we face. Some say we have longer lives than our ancestors; this is not true. They lived long, happy, and healthy lives.

This was a substantial shift, since before agriculture; our diets comprised vegetables, fruits, nuts, roots, and many types of meat (including vitamin rich organ meats, which are now often shunned). Although our cavemen ancestors might have consumed wild grains too, they would have done so sparingly.

Farming also suffers from the pesticides and organic sprays to enhance productivity, without knowing they are reducing the natural nutrients and allowing us to domesticate wild animals and feed them a grain-based diet, while their wild relatives would have thrived off grass.

Unfortunately, a grain-based diet for farm animals not only changes the taste of their meat, but it also modifies the quality of the proteins and fats found in the meat.

If we compare the meat obtained from grain fed animals to that obtained from grass-fed meat, we see the latter is much leaner, with lower amounts of saturated fats.

Grass-fed meat is also richer in heart healthy Omega-3 fats, when compared to the meat of grain fed animals, and infinitely more flavorful. One study that looked at the fatty acid contents found in meat sourced from wild deer and elk, concluded free range meat is far superior to grain fed meat and free range meat consumption may play a vital role in combating chronic disease in modern humans!

Studies also show that, ages ago, people never had cholesterol. The intake of rich fiber kept the cholesterol level in the body to the amount it caused no damage.

Now, with the modern diet, our bodies have preserved extra amounts of cholesterol, more than the requirement, because our fiber intake has gone low. No wonder most causes of deaths are related to heart diseases.

But grains and meat aren't the only problem with how we eat today, even when we're trying to eat healthy. Many dieticians are now comparing the standards of food quality between the ones that our ancestors used to consume and the food available right now.

Today's life is faster, which means we don't have time to invest in our diet routines. If we try to invest time, we realize how deteriorated our health has become. These days, our intake mainly includes processed fast food, not a proper intake of fruits and vegetables. Results? Low fibers in our body and diseases like constipation, cancers, obesity, heart diseases, and many others. Many diets recommend we cut back on processed foods and sugary drinks, as we focus on eating more fruits and vegetables.

The paleo diet takes this notion further, paying special attention to food source.

Where does your food come from and how was it grown? Is it wild, free range, or homegrown? Or is it commercially farmed? More scientific evidence suggests the quality of industrially grown fruits and vegetables has been declining steadily over the past hundred years, and the more we focus on industrial farming, the worse it will get.

Not only is industrial farming hurting our environment, but it is also hurting us. Genetically engineered food is not natural. It is a laboratory product.

Add to this the ubiquity of modern processed foods, like chips, microwave meals, cold meats, sugary deserts, pasta, soft drinks, and dairy products, and it's easy to see how our diets are working against us.

The biggest drawback of consuming the modern diet is that we age early. Our bodies are not formed to consume food against nature. Our bodies are also nature and the natural and artificial compatibility is equivalent to zero. With this in mind, all it takes is a conscious filter of all food we come across to ask if this food is as close to the source as possible.

Newly introduced foods during the Neolithic, Industrial, and modern eras are discordant with our species' ancient and conservative genome and can result in illness and disease. The adverse effects that cause diseases and early aging lower our standard of living.

A grim truth is that we are working so hard in our busy lives just to lower our standard of living. The return to center seems to have a large effect on our happiness in all aspects. In a way, the concept of Paleo, in that it goes back to the origin, is also a common line of reasoning in the niche of self-development and looking inside for answers.

How Going Paleo Can Boost Your Health

Whether you're struggling with unwanted weight, high cholesterol levels, elevated blood pressure, or chronic pain, science continuously shows the paleo diet can help you achieve the best results, while infusing you with essential nutrients that may be absent from traditional "healthy" diets.

What Is The Paleo Diet?

Several studies conducted in the past decade have demonstrated the paleo diet is more satiating per calorie, compared to both the Mediterranean diet and the standard recommended diet for diabetes. This means you can lose weight effortlessly, simply by eating until you're full.

Another study focused on weight loss pointed out it was impossible to stop a group of people on a paleo diet from losing weight, even when the research team topped off their daily menus with snacks. This same study concluded that being on a paleo diet for just two weeks improves several cardiovascular risk factors, compared to a healthy reference diet in patients suffering from metabolic syndrome.

Yet another study, which looked at the health benefits of a paleo diet for postmenopausal women, concluded it has long-term benefits, regarding abdominal obesity and triglyceride levels. In this study, the diet the women were on comprised lean meat, fish, eggs, vegetables, fruits, berries, and nuts. Cholesterol profiles for both men and women have also been shown to improve more dramatically on a paleo diet than on a standard "healthy" diet, based on whole grains.

The seven keys of a paleo diet:

i. Eat a higher amount of animal protein than that of an American diet, for example, beef, mutton, chicken, fish, turkey, al kind of sea food, bacon, steaks, and shrimp etc.

ii. Eat good amount of carbohydrates from fruits and vegetable not from today's typical process carbohydrate, starchy tuber, grains, and refined sugar.

iii. Take larger amount of fiber from non-starchy fruits and vegetables.

iv. Eat lower amount of monounsaturated and poly-saturated fat than saturated process fat.

v. Eat food containing low sodium and high potassium content.

vi. Make net alkaline load part of your paleo diet.

vii. Eat food, which contains a high amount of vitamins, minerals, and antioxidants. Plants rich in phytochemical should be the part of the paleo diet.

Okay, so if we cut out the grains, almost all processed foods, and dairy, you're left with only things that occur naturally:

- **Meat** – Grass-fed, not grain-fed. Grain causes the same problem in animals as they do in humans.

- **Fowl** – Chicken, duck, hen, turkey...things with wings that (try to) fly.

- **Fish** – Wild fish, as mercury and other toxins can be an issue in farmed fish.

- **Eggs** – Look for Omega-3 enriched eggs.

- **Vegetables** – As long as they're not deep-fried, eat as many as you want. Loaded with vitamins, minerals, fiber, fills you up. Doesn't spike your insulin and balances the acid-base (more alkaline as opposed to acidic).

- **Oils** – Olive oil, coconut oil, avocado oil – think natural.

- Fat ratios of omega 3/6/9, get normalized, and get more 3 w/ fish oil and more 9 w/ olive oil.

- **Fruits** – Have natural sugar and can be higher in calories, so limit if you're trying to lose weight. Fruits are still very good for you, naturally sweet, and loaded w/ nutrients. Keep your fruit intake less than vegetables.

- **Nuts** – High in calories, so they're good for a snack, but don't eat bags and bags. Anti-inflammatory.

- **Tubers** – Sweet potato and yam. Higher in calories and carbs, so these are good for right after a workout to replenish your glycogen levels.

Eating Paleo Is Beginner-Friendly

Because it is not based on familiar food items, like grains, legumes, or dairy, the paleo diet sometimes gets a bad rap for being hard to follow. Nothing could be farther from the truth!

Simply by changing how you prepare your food, you can turn some of your favorite old-school recipes into paleo goodness. The concept of the paleo diet is new to our generation, so we need to realize how important your health is and how careless we are about our daily meals, decaying our bodies in sweet manner.

Our daily routine is becoming so busy and fast we do not even bother about what we are eating. When we tell people about the paleo diet, they show reservation, and they do not want to change their diet routine, because they are addicted to the processed canned food.

If you're new to cooking or can't dedicate hours of your day to food preparation, then this is the perfect diet for you, because the beauty of eating paleo is found in its simplicity. Since this eating regimen is inspired by the diets of our ancestors, preparation methods are usually simple and don't call for any fancy tools or techniques.

Many people find the paleo diet can help improve blood lipids, reduce pain in autoimmunity, and weight loss. Some people blindly follow the paleo diet on someone's recommendation and can't get good results because they are not taking the proper paleo diet and adding another diet, according to what they are used to.

If you want to improve your health, you want to take a shift from your odd diet to acquiring more vitamins, minerals, and antioxidants. Also, know your requirement and ration of protein, fat, and carbohydrates.

Paleo diet includes high omega-3 acids and low omega -6 acids. Omega-3 acids can improve neurological function, reduce inflammation, restore healthy skin, improve focus, and help in digestion. Paleo experts say 60% of food should be gained from animals and 40% should be gained from fruits, vegetables, nuts, and seeds.

You can enjoy quick and easy folded omelets for breakfast, nuts, seeds, and fruits for snacks, poached salmon or luscious burgers for lunch, and juicy steaks with grilled vegetables for dinner!

Criticism And Different Interpretations

If you've been interested in health and nutrition for a while, chances are you've heard a lot of the criticism leveled at the paleo diet - our ancestors had a much shorter life span, eating paleo is expensive, or there is no consensus on what our prehistoric ancestors really ate, so we shouldn't make guesses.

While primitive humans had much shorter life spans on average than modern humans (many only lived for 30 to 40 years), this had less to do with what they ate and more to do with their hunter - gatherer lifestyle and the harsh conditions they lived in.

In prehistoric times, there were no hospitals, no supermarkets, and no central heating or hygiene, so infant mortality rates were high, and some cavemen could not survive into old age.

Conventional food and organic food are the main difference between us and our ancestors. Organic food is prepared according to standard, without considering the requirements, taste, and nutrient value. Some says organic food is good, but not always. In some scenarios, organic food is beneficial.

That doesn't mean an organic donut is good for you; it is still a donut, which is not good for you. Meat obtained from animals may be on antibiotic and growth hormones. Caged/farmed animals are given organic diet to gain maximum productivity, but still they cannot match the animal meat which gaze in greenery and wild ranges. They eat what they are meant to eat naturally.

Our ancestors would regularly fall prey to predators or disease, which contributed to their dismal life expectancy figures. We also need to consider that life expectancy figures are a mathematical average, so if infant mortality is high, it is going to skew the data dramatically.

It doesn't mean most people only lived to be 35, or that any lived to only 35. It just means infant mortality was high enough to reduce drastically the average lifespan you obtain on paper.

We do, however, have archaeological evidence that some cavemen lived well into old age. The skull of a 50,000-year-old Neanderthal man found in a small cave in France showed many signs of old age, leading scientists to believe he was in his 70s when he died.

If you remove infant mortality from the equation, the data suggests prehistoric humans lived comparably long lives to modern humans.

Because the paleo diet comprises high quality, nutrient rich foods, it is often perceived as expensive. Low quality, industrialized foods pumped with mass produced additives will always be cheaper, but is that really the food we want to put in our bodies?

Government surveys show the price of food has dropped a whopping 82% in the United States in the last century, thanks to industrialized agriculture (which has also made it possible to grain feed livestock), government subsidies encouraging cheaper production, and the fierce competition between giant food corporations.

If you look at the recommendations of a paleo diet, you might wonder why grass fed meat is more expensive, since grass grows naturally, and it should be free.

The explanation is simply that industrial livestock production is cost efficient and feeding animals corn is cheap; it allows food corporations to undercut the cost of growing grass-fed meat and sustainable farming.

Even though there are several takes on the paleo diet, the good news is they're likely all equally valid. Our stone-age ancestors were opportunistic and flexible eaters, and what they ate depended largely on what foods were available in their environment.

This means groups of cavemen in different parts of the world would have eaten very different foods.

Some paleo eaters exclude butter or vegetable oils entirely, while others believe these fats have a place in the paleo diet, even though they don't need to be consumed every day.

Sweeteners, such as honey or maple syrup, are also sometimes controversial, but since they are entirely naturally occurring foods that people have consumed for a long time, they can be considered paleo.

Organic red wine is also sometimes accepted by paleo eaters, though it is an indulgence; it is rich in antioxidants and nutrients. Non-gluten grains, such as brown rice, have made their way into more modern interpretations of the paleo diet, as has dark chocolate (which is also rich in free radical-fighting antioxidants).

The best general rule to follow when considering whether something is or isn't paleo is to ask yourself if the food occurs naturally. If it can be found in nature and is not processed or the result of industrial agriculture, then it is likely that stone-age humans ate it too.

Always listen to your body - if a certain food doesn't work for you, don't force yourself to eat it; our ancestors wouldn't have done it either.

Paleo Essentials:
What To Eat And What To Avoid

Now that we know the reasoning behind the Paleo diet. While preparing a meal, keep things simple. The simpler the meal is, the more paleo it's likely to be. Why is the paleo diet preferred over most other weight loss strategies? The answer is simple! Most other strategies involve complicated systems and tough charts to read and maintain.

While you are wrapped up in complications, the paleo diet helps you lose weight in the most unpretentious way possible. Since our bodies have a specific design and way of handling food for our benefit, we need a system that helps us by using nature to our benefit. Paleo diet is the most natural way of nurturing our body. It is not just a weight loss technique, but a way of pampering our body through the right use of nutrition and fiber.

Avoid adding chemicals, artificial flavors and make it free of additives. Eating paleo means eating meat, veggies, fish, fruits, nuts, seeds, and certain fats. The paleo list will become mouth drooling and next time, these items will be in your cart while grocery shopping. Let's take a quick look at the foods you should focus on, the foods you can eat in moderation, and the things you should absolutely avoid:

What you should not eat:

- All cereal grains, even whole meal and so-called "healthy" cereals (wheat and corn should be avoided, but also oats, rye and buckwheat) and any processed grain products, such as pasta and bread.

- Legumes, such as beans, peas, lentils, soybeans, chickpeas, and peanuts.

- Refined sugar and any sugary foods: table sugar, high fructose corn syrup, non-Paleo desserts, and soft drinks.

- Milk and dairy products: adults need not consume milk and most of us are lactose intolerant. Butter, cheese, or yogurt were not part of our ancestral diet.

- White potatoes: they're a starchy vegetable with a high glycemic index. While they're a natural food, our ancestors did not eat them, as they only became popular with agriculture.

- Vegetable seed oils.

- Table salt: ancestral diets were high in potassium and low in sodium.

- Any processed foods: including processed meats, canned products, trans-fats (margarine, hydrogenated oil), artificial sweeteners, any commercially available snack foods.

What you can eat, but only in moderation:

- Nuts and seeds - an important source of nutrients, but they are high in fat, and our ancestors consumed them sparingly.

- Fruits - they are high in fructose (fruit sugar), so try not to eat over 2 or 3 servings per day.

- Salt & spices - turmeric, rosemary, thyme, etc.

What you should eat

- All types of free range or wild meat, fish, and eggs - poultry, beef, lamb, turkey, quail, rabbit, wild boar, and even turtle. Fatty fish, such as salmon, is preferable, but you can also consume seafood, such as crab, lobster, clams, oysters, and shrimp.

- Organic or free range eggs.

- Oils and fats: avocado oil, coconut oil, olive oil, lard, tallow.

- Nearly all vegetables, except legumes and potatoes: eggplants, avocado, broccoli, beets, tomatoes, garlic, root vegetables, spinach, sweet potatoes, zucchini.

- Organic honey and maple syrup - these are the preferred sweeteners in the paleo diet, because they are entirely naturally occurring.

Appetizers

- Nut and Olive plate.

- Salad of organic, non-GMO mixed greens and veggies.

Nuts and seeds, both healthy fats, were a big part of the Paleolithic diet, as were weeds and vegetables. They likely found olives, too, says Steven Masley, M.D., author of *The 30 Day Heart Tune-Up*.

Entree

- Free range, grass-fed wild boar cooked in animal fat.

Animal protein in a paleo eating plan should be lean and clean. Most people just say, 'Hey, I'm doing paleo' as they chow down on bacon, hamburgers, chicken nuggets, and skip the bread, but this is hardly the case.

The diet excludes fatty cuts of meat and animal protein fattened on grain. Wild fish, deer, and elk are all on the menu, but grain-fed beef and pork are not. Pheasant, wild turkey, chukar, dove, quail, and other wild birds are acceptable, while hormone, pesticide-enriched chicken is a big no-no.

Dessert

- Berries sweetened with honey.

Our prehistoric ancestors didn't eat grains. They seldom had sugar, although some honey occasionally was an exciting find, says Masley. And don't even think about an after-dinner aperitif, as our ancestors didn't have alcohol.

"Considering that most people drink alcohol in excess, meaning more than one serving per day if they drink, all the alcohol just gets converted into sugar," he says.

The Dairy and Grain Debate

What about the issues with dairy and grains? Some proponents surrounding the diet center on excluding the two food groups entirely, which others would mention, leaves a nutritional hole that cannot be replaced easily. They also add the exclusion leaves out highly sought foods like yogurt, quinoa, beans, and whole grain oats.

Missing delicious and nutritious foods? Possibly. Nutritionally unbalanced? Not exactly. Experts say excluding grain and dairy increases the trace nutrient (vitamin, mineral, and phytochemical) density in your diet because of the simple fact that fresh vegetables, fruits, seafood, fish, and grass produced meat and poultry contain greater vitamins and minerals overall than grains and dairy.

Staying On Track:
4 Key Tips To Keep Your
Motivation Up

Picking up a new diet is easy, but what is often most difficult is ensuring you can adhere to it for the rest of your life. That means the changes you make to your lifestyle should be healthful, sustainable, and enjoyable.

Although this sounds easier said than done, do not be discouraged!

There are some tried and tested things you can do and some other things you should avoid doing to maximize your chances of success.

1. Take small, smart steps

One of the most common mistakes new dieters do is jump straight into their chosen diet from day one. While this sounds like a good idea at first, it rarely works in the long run, because you never gave yourself time to become accustomed to the particularities of your new diet. Making sudden, dramatic changes can be a shock for your body, and it is never a healthful option.

Instead, try making small changes you can keep track of. Give yourself a few days (or even a few weeks) to become accustomed to what you have changed. This also gives your body the time it needs to come off some substances it might have been addicted to, like sugar and artificial additives. When you take out one type of food, bring something healthful in.

This way, you won't feel like your new regimen is asking you to be restrictive, without giving you anything back.

No one is rushing you. Eating paleo isn't a competition, so give yourself all the time you need to do it right!

2. Listen to your body

...because it will tell you what it needs. Unfortunately, we are all different, so there is no perfect meal plan out there that can satisfy the dietary requirements of every person on the planet. That is why it is important to pay attention to your body and discover what works best for you.

Experiment with new foods and recipes whenever you can. Some people can get away with a light breakfast and a cup of coffee, while others need a hearty breakfast and an even more substantial lunch. Our ancestors did not have the privilege of modern medicine and blood tests, so they had to rely on their gut feelings about what they should eat. And it served them well for the most part.

You might also discover you are suddenly craving a specific food, which some scientists speculate is one of your body's ancestral ways of signaling a nutrient shortage. You might also find some foods make you uncomfortable or you're not enjoying them.

The paleo diet is about being creative and finding what best suits your needs.

3. Expect difficulty

Unfortunately, as much as we would like it to be perfect, no change-of-lifestyle process will be peaches and rainbows all the time. It's normal to feel demotivated on some days, to have a rough time when you struggle to stay on your paleo diet, or even to fall off track. It happens to everyone, and it doesn't mean you should give up and revert to your old diet.

Instead, go back to the basics and give yourself time to learn from your experience. You might discover you are having a much easier time with it on a second or third try, because you know what to expect and you know why it didn't work the first time around. Instead of viewing it as a failure, think of it as a learning experience that has enabled you to know yourself a little bit better.

4. Treat yourself!

Sometimes, having a healthy lifestyle can feel like it's all about what you can no longer do. This can lead to a vicious circle of negative reinforcement that will quickly undermine your motivation to press on. A good way to break through this vicious circle is to set simple goals and treat yourself whenever you reach them. If you've successfully been on the paleo diet for a month, celebrate this achievement by grabbing that nice pair of shoes you wanted, getting a fancy manicure, or even a relaxing day at a spa.

It's important to do something pleasurable, but it's vital that your chosen reward has nothing to do with food. If you reward yourself by going off the paleo diet, say by eating a pizza or a box of chocolate chip cookies, you're subconsciously telling yourself that eating paleo is something you endure until the next time you can go off it. It may seem like it is positive reinforcement, but in reality, it associates the paleo diet with frustration and the traditional diet with pleasure.

Paleo Recipes

Eating paleo is all about the simplicity and purity of flavors. Our ancestors didn't have advanced food preparation methods or complicated dishes, so the recipes you will find here are simple and can be easily whipped up, even if you are new to cooking!

Salads

Brussels Sprout, Raisin, And Apple Salad

Serves 4

Ingredients:

- 2 cups of Brussels sprouts, thinly sliced

- 1 medium red onion, finely julienned

- 2 Tbsp. Olive oil

- 1 cup chopped Pecan nuts

- 1 cup hemp seeds

- 1/2 cup raisins

- 1 red apple, cut to bite size

- 1 Tbsp. Lemon juice

- Salt & pepper to taste

Directions:

1. In a pan, heat the olive oil over medium heat and lightly cook the onion until golden.

2. Toss in the sliced Brussels sprouts and cook for a few minutes until tender.

3. Remove the pan from the heat and, as the brussel sprouts are cooling a bit, stir in the Pecan nuts, hemp seeds, apple and raisins.

4. Season with salt, pepper and lemon juice, and serve warm.

Avocado And Egg Salad

Serves 2

Ingredients:

- 6 hard boiled eggs
- 1 small red bell pepper, diced
- 1 avocado, diced
- 1 small red onion, diced
- 3 Tbsp mayonnaise
- 3 Tbsp chives, finely chopped
- 1 Tbsp lemon juice (optional)
- Salt & pepper to taste

Directions:

1. Chop the hard boiled eggs into quarters and place them into a mixing bowl. Add in the diced bell pepper, avocado, and onion

2. In a separate small bowl, combined the mayo, chives, and lemon juice and then add them to the salad, mixing all the ingredients well. Season with salt & pepper and serve.

Zesty Papaya Boat Breakfast

Serves 2

Ingredients:

- 1 large ripe papaya, cut in half length-wise
- 1 banana, diced
- 1/2 cup pineapple, diced
- 1 mango, diced
- 2 Tbsp almond flakes
- 1 Tbsp chia seeds
- 1 lime, juiced
- 2 Tbsp honey

Directions:

1. Scoop out the seeds from the papaya halves and put them in a pestle and mortar. Add in the honey and lime and grind everything together into a thick paste.

2. Place the papaya halves onto plates, fill their center with the diced fruit, then drizzle the dressing on top.

3. Sprinkle almond flakes and chia seeds for added texture and flavor and serve.

Chunky Salmon And Coconut Salad

Serves 2

Ingredients:

- 2 salmon fillets

- 1 Tbsp extra-virgin olive oil

- 1 teaspoon honey

- 1 Tbsp coconut sauce (raw, organic aminos or home-made)

- 1 romaine lettuce, chopped roughly

- 1 handful baby spinach

- 1 cup cucumber, sliced

- 1 avocado, sliced

- Salt & pepper to taste

Directions:

1. Heat the olive oil in a pan and fry the salmon fillets for 3 minutes on each side, until the skin is golden and they are cooked all the way through.

2. In a small bowl, mix the coconut sauce, honey, salt and pepper.

3. Spread the lettuce and the baby spinach onto two deep plates, and place the salmon fillets on top.

4. Toss the avocado and cucumber slices around the salmon and drizzle the coconut and honey dressing on top. Serve warm.

Tomato And Spinach Salad

Serves 4

Ingredients:

- 4 yellow tomatoes, cut into wedges

- 8 oz. grape tomatoes, halved

- 8 oz. baby spinach leaves

- ¼ cup toasted pine nuts

- ¼ cup fresh basil, coarsely chopped

- ¼ cup extra-virgin <u>olive oil</u>

- 2 tbsp. balsamic vinegar

- Sea salt and freshly ground black pepper

Directions:

1. Combine the olive oil and balsamic vinegar in a bowl.

2. Stir until well combined and season to taste.

3. Combine the tomatoes, basil, spinach, and pine nuts in a large bowl.

4. Drizzle the dressing on top, and toss gently to combine

Creamy Cucumber Salad Recipe

Serves 4

Ingredients:

- 1 lb. cucumber, sliced;
- ¼ cup homemade <u>mayonnaise</u>;
- 1 tbsp. fresh dill, finely chopped;
- 1 tbsp. fresh chives, finely chopped;
- 1 tbsp. white wine <u>vinegar</u>;
- Sea salt and freshly ground black pepper

Directions:

1. In a large bowl, combine the mayonnaise, dill, chives, vinegar, and season to taste with salt and pepper. Mix well.

2. Add the cucumber slices to the bowl, and stir gently until everything is combined.

3. Refrigerate or serve right away.

Fruit Salad

Serves 2

Ingredients:

- ½ cup pineapple, diced

- 1 kiwi fruit, diced

- 1 small banana chopped

- ½ cup mango, diced

- 4 lychees, seeds removed

- ½ cup green grapes, seeds removed

- 1 passion fruit pulp

Directions:

1. Combine all ingredients into a medium sized mixing bowl.

Thai Ground Chicken Salad

Serves 4

Ingredients:

- 2 Tbsp. lime juice, preferably fresh squeezed
- 2 tsp minced fresh ginger
- 1 tsp honey
- 1/8 tsp chili garlic sauce, or to taste
- 1/8 tsp salt
- 1 ½ tsp extra-virgin olive oil
- 1/4-pound extra-lean ground chicken
- 2 cups shredded romaine lettuce leaves
- ½ cup shredded carrot
- ¼ cup red onion slivers
- 2Tbsp chopped fresh mint leaves
- 1 Tbsp. chopped fresh cilantro leaves
- 1 to 2 Tbsp. chopped dry-roasted cashews

Directions:

1. In a small bowl, combine the lime juice, ginger, honey, chili garlic sauce, and salt. Whisk, gradually adding the oil, until blended.

2. Set a small nonstick frying pan over medium-high heat until it is hot enough for a spritz of water to sizzle on it.

3. With an oven mitt, briefly remove the pan from the heat to lightly mist with olive oil spray.

4. Add the chicken to the pan.

5. Cook, breaking up the meat into chunks with a spatula, for 3 to 5 minutes, or until no longer pink.

6. Remove from the heat and stir in 1 tablespoon of the reserved dressing.

7. In a large serving bowl, combine the lettuce, carrot, onion, mint, and cilantro.

8. Drizzle with the remaining dressing and toss.

9. Top with reserved chicken and sprinkle with the nuts.

10. Serve immediately.

Soups

Sweet Potato And Pear Cream Soup

Serves 4

Ingredients:

- 2 large sweet potatoes, peeled and chopped
- 2 pears, peeled and chopped
- 1 cup turnip, peeled and chopped
- 1 red onion, minced
- 4 cups chicken or vegetable stock
- 4 Tbsp coconut milk
- 1/2 Tbsp curry powder
- 1 Tbsp extra-virgin olive oil
- A handful of chives, minced
- Salt & pepper to taste

Directions:

1. In a sauce pan, heat the olive oil over medium heat and sauté the minced onion until translucent.

2. Add in the chopped sweet potatoes, pears and turnips and cook for about 5 minutes, stirring often.

3. Pour in the chicken or vegetable stock and bring everything to a boil.

4. Cover the saucepan, turn the heat down a bit and cook for about 25 minutes.

5. Remove from heat source and puree the soup until you smooth and then add in the coconut milk, curry powder, salt and pepper, and mix everything together.

6. Garnish each soup bowl with fresh chives and serve warm.

Quick Chicken And Leek Soup

Serves 4

Ingredients:

- 1 large leek, finely sliced
- 1 large cooked chicken breast (oven baked is best)
- 2 garlic cloves, minced
- 5 cups chicken stock
- 1/2 cup coconut milk
- 2 Tbsp coconut oil
- A handful of parsley, roughly chopped (optional)
- Salt & pepper to taste

Directions:

1. Melt the coconut oil in a large pan, over medium heat.
2. Add the leeks and cook them until soft, about 10 minutes (be careful not to over-cook them).
3. Add the chicken stock and bring to a boil, stirring frequently.
4. Turn the heat down to low and let it simmer for about 15 minutes.
5. Add the cooked chicken and coconut milk and cook for about 5 more minutes.

6. Season with salt and pepper and serve warm, garnished with parsley.

Winter Gizzard Soup

Serves 4

Ingredients:

- 2 lbs chicken gizzards

- 3 medium sized zucchini, sliced

- 1 red bell pepper, sliced

- 2 parsnips, peeled and chopped

- 4 garlic cloves, minced

- 1 small leek, finely sliced

- 3 cups beef or vegetable broth

- 3 cups water

- 1 Tbsp. lard (or bacon fat)

- Salt & pepper to taste

Directions:

1. Melt the lard in a deep saucepan, toss in the gizzards and allow them to brown for about 10 minutes.

2. While the gizzards are cooking, chop and slice the zucchini, parsnip, leek, garlic, and bell pepper.

3. Add all your vegetables to the pot and cook together, stirring continuously for about 2 minutes.

4. Add the broth and water, bring everything to boil, cover the pot, and let the soup simmer over low heat for about 1 hour.

5. Season with salt and pepper and serve warm.

Spaghetti Squash Noodle And Meatball Soup

Serves 4

Ingredients:

<u>For the meatballs:</u>

- 1 lb ground beef
- 1 small yellow onion, very finely chopped
- 2 Tbsp unsalted butter
- 1 Tbsp parsley, finely chopped
- 1 whole egg
- Salt & pepper to taste

<u>For the soup:</u>

- 8 cups chicken, beef or vegetable broth
- 1 medium spaghetti squash
- 4 white button mushrooms, finely sliced
- 1 small yellow onion, chopped
- 1 medium carrot, peeled and chopped
- Salt & pepper to taste

Directions:

1. To prepare the spaghetti squash, cut it in half lengthwise and remove its seeds.

2. Place the 2 pieces cut side down on a baking tray and bake at 350 degrees, for about 40 minutes (or until tender).

3. In a small pan, melt the butter and cook the onion for the meatballs for a few minutes, until soft and translucent.

4. In a mixing bowl, combine the ground meat, sautéed onion, chopped parsley, egg and seasoning and mix them together thoroughly.

5. Bring 2 cups of broth to a simmer in a large pot.

6. Start forming small meatballs (about 1 teaspoon of meat) and drop them into the simmering broth and cook for a few minutes, until they're almost done.

7. Add the remaining 6 cups of broth, the mushrooms, chopped onion and carrot to the simmering pot.

8. Let everything cook together until done, about 20-25 minutes.

9. Ladle the soup into serving bowls and serve with spaghetti squash. Do not add the spaghetti squash directly into the pot because it can quickly overcook and lose its texture.

Meatball Minestrone Soup

Serves 2

Ingredients:

- 1 tbsp. oil

- 1 onion, diced

- 3 garlic cloves, finely chopped

- ¼ white cabbage, thinly sliced

- 2 medium carrots, diced

- 3 small zucchini, diced

- 3 celery stalks, diced

- 14.5 oz. can dice tomatoes or 1½ cups diced tomatoes

- 3 cups chicken or vegetable stock

- 1 tbsp. basil, finely chopped

- 1 tbsp. sage, finely chopped

- 1 tsp Mexican chili powder

- Dash pepper

- 2 cups mushroom, diced

Directions:

1. In a large pan on medium heat fry onion and garlic in oil until browned.

2. Add cabbage, carrots, zucchini, celery, tomatoes, stock, basil, sage, chili powder and pepper. Cover and boil for 30 minutes.

3. Add mushrooms and meatballs and cook for a further 10 minutes.

4. Leave to cool for 5-10 minutes before serving.

Main Dishes

Slow Cooked Butternut Squash And Beef Stew

Serves 4

Ingredients:

- 1 lb beef, cubed
- 1 butternut squash, de-seeded, peeled and diced
- 1 medium yellow onion, diced
- 3 garlic cloves, minced
- 1 cup mushrooms, sliced
- 1 cup spinach, roughly chopped
- 1 cup chicken or vegetable stock
- 2 cups plum tomatoes, diced
- 1 teaspoon paprika
- 1 teaspoon chili powder
- 1 teaspoon dried oregano
- Handful of fresh parsley, chopped (optional)
- 1 Tbsp lard
- Salt & pepper to taste

Directions

1. In a deep pan, brown the beef cubes in olive oil for about 2 minutes.

2. Add the squash, onion, tomatoes, stock, herbs and spices, and cover the pot. Let everything cook slowly, either over very low heat or in the oven, for about 5 hours.

3. Just 30 minutes before the stew is done, add in the mushrooms and garlic. 2 minutes before turning the heat off completely, add in the spinach and give everything a good stir.

4. Adjust with salt and pepper, sprinkle with parsley and serve!

Egg And Pesto Stuffed Tomatoes

Serves 2

Ingredients:

- 6 large tomatoes

- 6 eggs

- 6 romaine lettuce leaves

- 1/2 cup extra-virgin olive oil

- 1 large garlic clove

- a handful of cilantro

- 1/4 teaspoon oregano

- Salt & pepper to taste

Directions:

For the pesto:

1. Add the lettuce leaves, garlic, cilantro, oregano, olive oil, salt and pepper to a blender and process until the pesto reaches the desired consistency.

2. If the pesto is not thick enough or doesn't hold together well, add 2 more lettuce leaves and a bit more olive oil.

For the stuffed tomatoes:

1. Preheat your oven to 400 F.

2. Using a vegetable knife or a spoon, scoop out the pulp and the seeds from the tomatoes.

3. Place the tomatoes face up on a baking tray, and fill them with pesto just a bit more than half way through, making sure you leave enough space in each for the egg.

4. Crack the eggs and add one in each tomato.

5. Season with salt and pepper and roast the stuffed tomatoes in the pre-heated oven for about 20 to 25 minutes.

6. Serve immediately!

Sesame Spiced Tuna Steak

Serves 4

Ingredients:

- 4 large tuna steaks
- 1 teaspoon mustard seeds
- 4 Tbsp sesame seeds
- 1 teaspoon fennel seeds
- 3 Tbsp coconut oil
- Salt & black pepper to taste

Directions:

1. Mix the fennel seeds, mustard seeds, the salt and the pepper in a mortar, and grind everything together coarsely.

2. Transfer the ground seeds into a small bowl, and mix in the sesame.

3. Spread the spices on a plate, and press each tuna steak into the mixture, allowing them to coat evenly on both sides.

4. In a frying pan, melt the coconut oil over medium heat and cook each tuna steak for 3 minutes on each side (about 6 or 7 minutes in total).

5. Serve immediately as is or accompanied by a light salad.

Paleo Recipes

Meatball Bites With Spaghetti Squash Recipe

Serves 4

Ingredients:

- 2 spaghetti squash, cut in half lengthwise and seeds removed

- 1 lb. ground beef

- 4 egg whites, whisked

- 1 egg

- ½ tbsp. dried parsley

- ½ tbsp. dried basil

- ½ tbsp. dried thyme

- Paleo cooking fat

- Sea salt and freshly ground black pepper

Ingredients for the tomato sauce:

- 2 cups good quality tomato sauce;

- 1 garlic clove, minced;

- ½ tbsp. dried parsley;

- ½ tbsp. dried basil;

- ½ tbsp. dried thyme;

- Sea salt and freshly ground black pepper

Directions:

1. Preheat your oven to 425 F.

2. Place the spaghetti squash on a baking sheet, cut side down, and bake for 25 to 30 minutes.

3. Combine the ground beef, dried parsley, dried, basil, dried thyme, and egg, and season to taste with salt and pepper.

4. Mix everything until well combined.

5. Roll the meat into meatballs of about 1 inch in diameter.

6. In a bowl, combine all the ingredients for the tomato sauce and season to taste.

7. In a large skillet placed over a medium heat, sauté the meatballs until browned on all sides.

8. Add the tomato sauce to the skillet and cook for 7 to 10 minutes, or until the meatballs are cooked through.

9. Once the spaghetti squash is cooked, use a large spoon to scoop the stringy pulp from the squash and place in a bowl.

10. Lower the oven's heat to 350 F.

11. Mix the egg white with the spaghetti squash, and then fill each cavity of a muffin tin with the squash mix, pressing down in the middle to make a "nest" for the meatball.

12. Place one meatball on top of each muffin and place in the oven for about 15 minutes.

13. Serve with remaining sauce drizzled on top of each meatball bite.

Tuna Burger

Serves 4

Ingredients:

- 1 lb. fresh tuna, diced

- 2 scallions, thinly sliced

- 12 Kalamata olives, pitted and chopped

- ¼ cup homemade mayonnaise

- 1 tsp. anchovy paste

- Extra-virgin olive oil, for brushing

- Sliced tomatoes and arugula, to serve

- Sea salt and freshly ground black pepper, to taste

Directions:

1. Preheat your grill to medium high.

2. In a bowl, combine the tuna, the Kalamata olives, and the scallions. Place the mixture in the freezer for 5 minutes.

3. When the 5 minutes is up, transfer the tuna mixture into a food processor and pulse until the tuna is finely chopped.

4. Transfer back to the bowl and season to taste.

5. Flatten the tuna into 4 patties of equal size.

6. Brush each patty with olive oil and grill for 6 to 8 minutes total, flipping once.

7. In a small bowl, combine the mayonnaise with the anchovy paste.

8. Spread the mayonnaise and anchovy paste on each tuna patty.

9. Top with tomato and arugula and serve.

Butter Chicken

Serves 4

Ingredients:

- 4 tbsp. of pastured, grass-fed butter

- About 1 kg chicken cut into chunks

- 2 tsp garam masala

- 2 tsp paprika

- 2 tsp ground coriander

- 1 tbsp. grated fresh ginger

- 1/4 tsp chili powder (adjust to taste)

- 1 cinnamon stick

- 6 bruised cardamon pods

- 1 can of tomato puree (you can easily puree your own tomatoes if they are meaty enough)

- 3/4 cup coconut milk

- 1 tbsp. fresh lemon juice

Directions:

1. Heat a pan, add the first 2 tbsp. of butter and stir-fry the chicken chunks. You can cook them in 2 batches if your pan is too small.

2. Remove the chicken from the pan.

3. Put the second 2 tbsp. of butter and slowly heat the spices for a minute or two until you can smell the aroma.

4. Put the chicken back in the pan and stir so you mix in all the spices with the chicken.

5. At this point, add the tomatoes and simmer for about 15 minutes. Stir from time to time.

6. Add the coconut milk and lemon juice and let it simmer for another 5 minutes.

7. Enjoy without guilt! Garnish with fresh herbs and a stick of cinnamon for extra fanciness points.

Frittatas

Serves 4

Ingredients

- 1 tbsp. choice of fat oil

- 1 cup emergency protein

- 1 cup frozen vegetables of choice (I'd prefer broccoli, carrots, onions and capsicum)

- 4 large or medium sized eggs

- 2 tbsp. coconut milk

- 1 tsp. salt

- ½ tsp. or to taste black pepper

Directions:

1. Heat the preferred oil in a cast iron pan over medium flame.

2. Add the emergency or left over protein into the oil and fry it till fully heated.

3. Place the vegetables of choice in a microwave safe bowl and heat it just enough that all the vegetables are damp and defrosted.

4. With a knife or kitchen shears, cut out the veggies down to bite size.

5. Add these veggies into the cast iron pan and mix them with mince till heated thoroughly.

6. Crack the eggs in a bowl and add coconut milk, salt and sprinkle black pepper into it.

7. Beat the eggs well so that all the ingredients in it also mix finely.

8. Add the egg mixture in a separate nonstick pan and heat just enough to make the frittata base out of it.

9. Add the mince mixture on the nonstick pan and insert it into the oven.

10. Keep the temperature to 350° F.

11. Once it is baked well, carefully place the frittata to a dish.

12. Sprinkle a little bit of black and white (optional) pepper and make slices.

13. After cooling down, serve it immediately.

Sides/Vegetables

Jalapeno Poppers Recipe

Serves 4

Ingredients:

- 10 jalapeno peppers, sliced in half and seeded
- 10 bacon slices, cut in half
- 10 mini sausages or full sausages sliced in 10 pieces
- 1 cup almond cheese (optional)
- 1 tsp. chili powder

Directions:

1. Preheat your oven to 425 F.

2. If using almond cheese, mix it with the chili powder in a bowl.

3. Fill each jalapeno cavity with the almond cheese.

4. Place a sausage on top of each jalapeno.

5. Wrap each popper with half a bacon slice and secure with a toothpick if needed.

6. Place on a baking sheet, and cook in the oven for 20 minutes.

7. Serve warm.

Cauliflower Tortillas Recipe

Serves 4

Ingredients:

- 1 head of cauliflower, cut up and stems removed

- 2 large eggs

- ½ tsp. dried oregano

- ½ tsp. paprika

- Sea salt and freshly ground black pepper

Directions:

1. Preheat your oven to 375 F.

2. Using a blender or a food processor, pulse the cauliflower until you get a texture finer than rice.

3. Steam the riced cauliflower over boiling water for 5 minutes.

4. Place the steamed cauliflower in a dish towel and squeeze out as much excess water as you can. You might want to let it cool for a few minutes first, so you don't burn yourself. You should be able to get out a lot of water; be really aggressive about squeezing it, or you'll end up with soggy tortillas later.

5. Transfer the cauliflower to a bowl. Add in the eggs, oregano, and paprika, and season to taste (you can use any spices you like).

6. Separate the mixture into 6 balls of equal size, and spread each ball out on a parchment-lined baking sheet to make six small circles.

7. Place in the oven and bake for 8 to 10 minutes; then flip and cook for another 5 minutes.

8. Reheat in a pan placed over low heat when ready to serve.

Carrot-Mushroom Stir-Fry

Serves 4

Ingredients:

- 6 carrots, sliced thin
- 4 tbsp olive oil
- 5 scallions, sliced into thin pieces
- 10 medium mushrooms, sliced thin
- 1 tbsp lemon juice
- ½ tsp black pepper

Directions:

1. Steam carrots until tender. Heat oil in large skillet.

2. Add carrots, scallions, and mushrooms and stir-fry until all are cooked.

3. Add lemon juice and pepper and mix well.

4. Serve and enjoy!

Mini Hamburger Bites Recipe

Serves 4

Ingredients:

- 1 1/2 lbs. ground beef
- 4 bacon slices, cooked
- 10 cherry tomatoes, halved
- 1 cup lettuce, chopped
- 4 pickles, sliced into 5 pieces each to make 20 discs
- Sea salt and freshly ground pepper

Directions:

1. Preheat a grill or griddle to medium-high.

2. Form 20 mini patties with the ground beef, and season each patty with sea salt and freshly ground black pepper.

3. Place the patties on a grill or griddle. Cook for 2 to 3 minutes per side and set aside.

4. To assemble the burger bites, top each patty with a piece of bacon, lettuce, pickle, and tomato.

5. Secure each patty with a toothpick, and serve with your favorite <u>condiments</u>.

Apple And Vegetable Stir-Fry

Serves 4

Ingredients:

- 1 head broccoli, cut into florets

- 1 cup onion, sliced

- 1 cup carrot, julienned

- 1 cup celery, sliced

- 1-2 apples, sliced

Cooking fat

Ingredients for the orange ginger sauce

- ½ cup fresh orange juice

- 2 tbsp. coconut aminos

- 2 tbsp. white wine vinegar

- 1 tbsp. fish sauce

- 1 tbsp. orange zest

- 2 garlic cloves, minced

- 1 thumb size piece of ginger, minced

Directions:

1. Combine all the ingredients for the sauce in a large bowl.

2. Heat a skillet over medium-high heat and melt some cooking fat.

3. Add the broccoli and carrot and cook until tender but still somewhat crunchy, about 5 minutes.

4. Add the onion and celery and cook for another 5 minutes.

5. Drizzle the sauce over the mixture, and cook for 2 to 3 minutes.

6. Add the apple, stir everything, cook for another 2 to 3 minutes, and serve.

Desserts

No-Bake Giant Nut Cookies

Serves 2

Ingredients:

- 6 Tbsp coconut flour, sifted

- 2 Tbsp almond flour

- 4 Tbsp maple syrup (or other sweetener of choice)

- 4 Tbsp crunchy almond butter (or other nut butter of choice)

- 2 Tbsp nut mix of choice (cashew and almonds work best)

- 1/4 teaspoon of cinnamon

- A pinch of salt

- 1/2 cup almond milk

Directions:

1. Take a large mixing bowl and combine the flours, cinnamon and salt.

2. Add in the nut butter and maple syrup and mix well, until you obtain a mixture with a thick and crumbly texture.

3. Start gently mixing in the almond milk, pouring 1 Tbsp at a time, until you obtain a very thick batter.

4. Using your hands, turn the batter into two large balls and then press them firmly against a plate to flatten them into a rough cookie shape.

5. Refrigerate the cookies for at least 30 minutes before serving.

6. Enjoy your delicious cookies!

Strawberry Crumble

Serves 4

Ingredients:

<u>For the filling:</u>

- 4 cups fresh strawberries, halved

- 2 Tbsp tapioca flour

- 2 teaspoons vanilla extract

- 1 Tbsp fresh lemon juice

- 2 Tbsp pure maple syrup

<u>For the crumble:</u>

- 1 cup almond flour

- A pinch of salt

- 3 Tbsp coconut oil

- 3 Tbsp maple syrup

Directions:

1. Preheat your oven to 350 F.

2. Take a large bowl and toss in the halved strawberries, tapioca flour, lemon juice, vanilla extract and 2 Tbsp of maple syrup.

3. Mix everything together well and transfer to a baking pan.

4. In a separate bowl, mix together the almond flour, salt, coconut oil and 3 Tbsp of maple syrup.

5. Spread this crumble evenly over the strawberry filling and bake for about 30 minutes, or until the topping has turned golden-brown.

6. Let the crumble cool for about 10 minutes.

7. Serve either as is or with a spoonful of ice cream!

Simple Banana Ice Cream

Serves 2

Ingredients:

- 3 large, ripe bananas
- 1 Tbsp coconut flakes
- a handful of chopped nuts (almond or cashews)

Directions:

1. Peel the bananas and cut them into even slices, about half an inch thick.

2. Put the banana slices in a glass bowl and let them cool in the freezer overnight.

3. Toss the frozen bananas into a blender or food processor, and process until you obtain a smooth cream. If the bananas stick to the food processor bowl, use a spatula to scrape down the sides.

4. Once the banana cream has reached the desired consistency, put it back into the bowl and freeze for at least an hour before serving.

5. Garnish with coconut flakes and chopped nuts and enjoy!

Apple And Almond Butter Bites

Serves 2

Ingredients:

- 1 red apple, cored and thinly sliced

- 1/2 cup almond butter (you might need to use more or less, depending on how many apple slices you have)

- A handful of pecan nuts, chopped

- A handful of almonds, sliced

- 2 Tbsp roasted coconut shreds

- 1/2 teaspoon cinnamon powder (optional)

- 2 Tbsp dried cranberries

Directions:

1. Spread the apple slices evenly on a platter.

2. Spread almond butter over each of the apple slices (make sure the butter layer isn't very thick).

3. Top each slices with a few pieces of pecans, almonds, cranberries and coconut shreds.

4. Sprinkle powdered cinnamon powder on top.

5. Serve it as a snack, dessert or breakfast!

Lemon Tarts

Serves 2

Ingredients:

<u>Pastry</u>

- 1 cup almond meal

- 3 tbsp. lemon juice

- 4 dates

<u>Filling</u>

- 6 tbsp. lemon juice

- 1 lemon, rind finely grated

- 1 tbsp. honey

- 2 eggs

Directions:

1. Pre -heat oven to 350 degrees Fahrenheit.

2. To make the pastry, place ingredients into a blender and mix until well combined. In a muffin tray (or similar) line individual holes with baking paper, and firmly place pastry mixture on the bottom and sides. Bake in oven for 10 -12 minutes, or until pastry has browned. Leave to cool.

3. To make the filling. Place lemon juice, lemon rind and honey into a pan, and simmer on low heat for 2 minutes. In a bowl, beat eggs well. Slowly add the

beaten eggs to simmering filling, stirring vigorously to form a nice smooth texture. Add more honey if desired. Leave to cool slightly.

4. When pastry has cooled, and the filling has reduced to a warm temperature, spoon the filling into each individual tart.

5. Place in the fridge until cooled and set. Makes around 4, depending on size.

6. Serve and enjoy!

Coconut Milk Ice Cream

Serves 4

Ingredients:

- 1 can coconut milk

- 2 cups fresh fruit

- 1 tsp vanilla (optional)

Directions:

This is an easy recipe that can be used to satisfy your hankering for a cool and refreshing dessert. We especially love using fresh strawberries, blueberries and peaches.

1. Simply place all ingredients in blender and puree.

2. Pour into dessert cups (coffee cups work equally well) and put in the freezer for about 1 hour or until it has chilled to an ice cream-like consistency.

Makes 4 cups Zone blocks: This is a fat intensive recipe, but listen, it's ice cream! One can of coconut milk (13.5 oz.) contains 45g or 30 blocks of fat. 2 Cups of berries is equal to 4 blocks of carbs. A one-cup serving of Coconut Milk ice cream yields 1 block carb, and about 7 blocks fat.

All these recipes are not just delicious dishes to be a part of a paleo diet routine, but they are also a good way of consuming the required fat, proteins and other nutrients into our system. People who say that they are "going Paleo" are in fact "going healthy". This is a complete lifestyle for all those people who want to adopt a healthy diet routine and be able to lose weight in no time.

Before You Go

If you liked this book, you may like these other popular books from **Jennifer Sullivan**

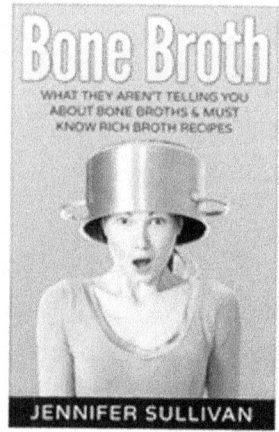 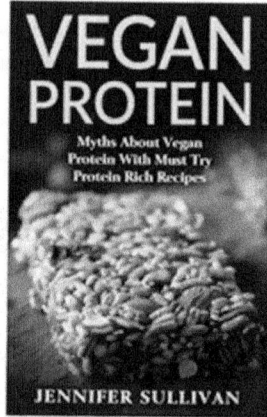 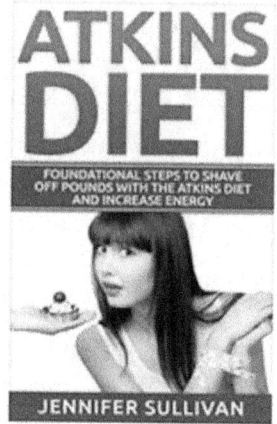

Check out more books from **Jennifer Sullivan**

>>Visit<<

https://www.amazon.com/Jennifer-Sullivan/e/B01J4O3N6U/

If you didn't download your **FREE** Gift to "**Habits: The Essential Guide**" yet you can get it by clicking below.

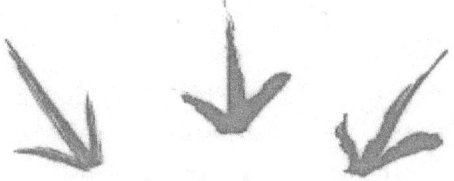

>>Visit The Link Below To Download "Habits: The Essential Guide" For FREE<<

https://cueballpublishing.leadpages.co/free-habits-ebook/

Conclusion

Thank you again for joining me on this journey!

I hope this book was able to help you learn more about the paleo diet with concrete actionable ideas. We should try to add more things that add value in our routine. The paleo diet is far better and healthier than our American diet. We should be more inclined toward natural foods rather than processed foods so commonly advertised. One must go and enjoy the best of natural foods!

The next step is to implement these strategies and share your paleo diet results with me and other people to motivate them as well!

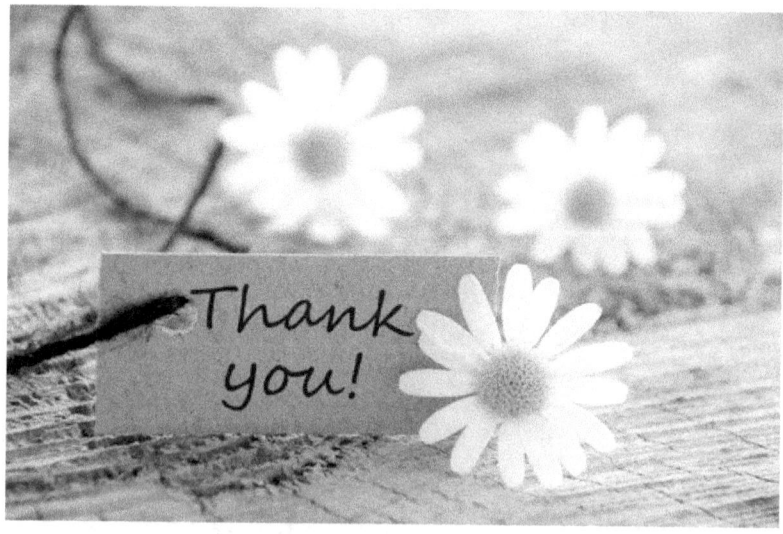

Finally, if you enjoyed this book, then I'd like to ask you for a favor, would you be kind enough to leave a review for this book on Amazon? It'd be greatly appreciated!

Thank you and good luck!

www.ingramcontent.com/pod-product-compliance
Lightning Source LLC
Chambersburg PA
CBHW062058280526
45788CB00003B/1273